C000132431

The Ultimate Vegetarian Sweet & Savory Recipe Book

Delicious Sweet And Savory
Vegetarian Dishes For Everyone

Adam Denton

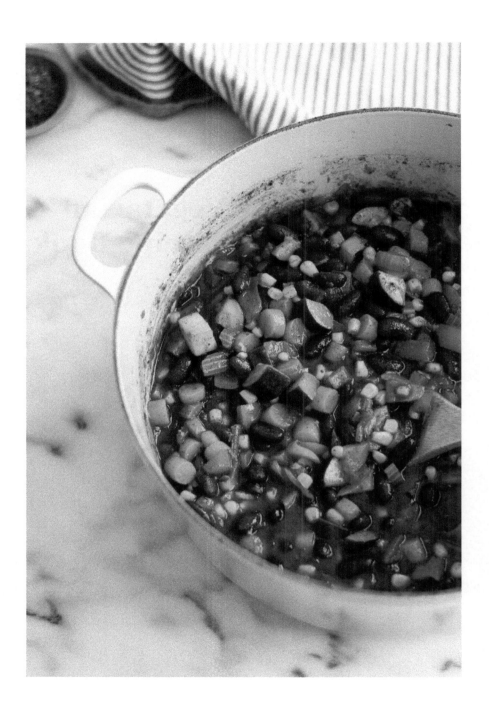

© Copyright 2020 - All rights reserved.

The content contained within this book may not be reproduced, duplicated or transmitted without direct written permission from the author or the publisher.

Under no circumstances will any blame or legal responsibility be held against the publisher, or author, for any damages, reparation, or monetary loss due to the information contained within this book. Either directly or indirectly.

Legal Notice:

This book is copyright protected. This book is only for personal use. You cannot amend, distribute, sell, use, quote or paraphrase any part, or the content within this book, without the consent of the author or publisher.

Disclaimer Notice:

Please note the information contained within this document is for educational and entertainment purposes only. All effort has been executed to present accurate, up to date, and reliable, complete information. No warranties of any kind are declared or implied. Readers acknowledge that the author is not engaging in the rendering of legal, financial, medical or professional advice. The content within this book has been derived from various sources. Please consult a licensed professional before attempting any techniques outlined in this book.

By reading this document, the reader agrees that under no circumstances is the author responsible for any losses, direct or indirect, which are incurred as a result of the use of information contained within this document, including, but not limited to, — errors, omissions, or inaccuracies.

Table of contents

Quick pitta pizzas

Prep: 10 mins

Cook: 10 mins

Easy

Serves 2

Ingredients

- 4 wholewheat pitta breads
- 4 tsp sun-dried tomato purée
- 3 ripe plum tomatoes , diced
- 1 shallot , thinly sliced
- 85g chorizo , diced
- 50g mature cheddar , grated
- few basil leaves , if you like

Directions:

1. Heat oven to 200C/180C fan/gas 6 and put a baking sheet inside to heat up. Spread each pitta with 1 tsp purée. Top with the tomatoes, shallot, chorizo and cheddar.

2. Place on the hot sheet and bake for 10 mins until the pittas are crisp, the cheese has melted and the chorizo has frazzled edges. Scatter with basil, if you like, and serve with a green salad.

Rainbow cookies

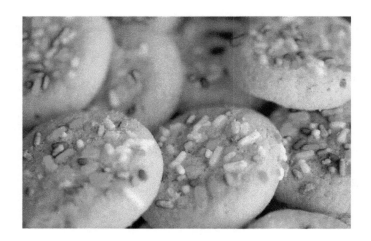

Prep: 25 mins - 30 mins

Cook:15 mins

Easy

Makes 22

Ingredients

- 175g softened butter
- 50g golden caster sugar
- 50g icing sugar
- 2 egg yolks
- 2 tsp vanilla extract

- 300g plain flour
- zest and juice 1 orange
- 140g icing sugar , sifted
- sprinkles , to decorate

Directions:

1. Heat oven to 200C/180C fan/gas 6. Mix the butter, sugars, egg yolks and vanilla with a wooden spoon until creamy, then mix in the flour in 2 batches. Stir in the orange zest. Roll the dough into about 22 walnut-size balls and sit on baking sheets. Bake for 15 mins until golden, then leave to cool.

2. Meanwhile, mix the icing sugar with enough orange juice to make a thick, runny icing. Dip each biscuit half into the icing, then straight into the sprinkles. Dry on a wire rack.

Apple 'doughnuts'

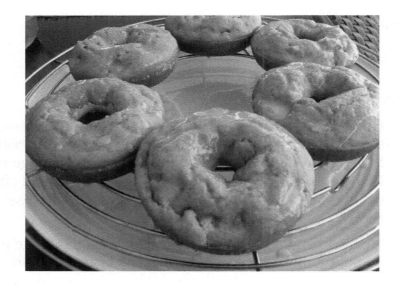

Prep: 20 mins

No cook

Easy

Makes 15

Ingredients

- 150g soft cheese
- 2 tsp honey
- 3 apples (use a crunchy eating variety)

- 3-4 tbsp almond or peanut butter (optional)
- coloured sprinkles , to decorate

Directions:

1. Mix the soft cheese with the honey and set aside. Peel the apples, then slice each through the core into five or six rings, about 1cm thick. Use an apple corer or small round biscuit cutter to stamp out a circle from the middle of each slice, removing the core and creating 'doughnut' shapes. Pat the slices dry using kitchen paper – they should be as dry as possible to help the toppings stick.

2. Spread some nut butter over the slices, if using, then top with the sweetened soft cheese. Decorate with the sprinkles and serve.

Cuddly egg men

Prep: 20 mins

Cook: 20 mins Plus rising

Easy

Makes 4

Ingredients

- 400g strong white flour
- ½ tsp salt
- pinch of sugar
- 7g sachet fast-action dried yeast
- 2 tbsp olive oil
- 4 large eggs , at room temperature

Directions:

1. Put the flour into a large bowl and stir in the salt, sugar and yeast. Pour in 250ml water and the oil and mix to a soft dough. Add a little extra water if necessary.

2. Knead the dough for a few minutes until smooth and then put into a bowl, cover and leave in a warm place for about 1 hour or until doubled in size.

3. Heat the oven to 200C/180C fan/gas 6. Turn the dough out onto a board, knead briefly and then cut into four. Take one piece and cut off a quarter and shape into a ball for the

head. Shape the other piece into a sausage. Attach the head to the body using a little cold water.

4. Place the dough onto a non-stick baking sheet. Using a sharp knife cut the bottom half of the sausage to make two legs, then cut into the sides up to the shoulders to make two arms. Using scissors, snip at intervals around the top of the head to make hair and make one snip for the mouth. Use a wooden skewer to make two eyes.

5. Take one egg and place on the dough man's tummy. Fold the arms over the egg and secure with a little cold water. Make three more egg men with the remaining dough. Leave to prove for about 10 mins.

6. Bake in the oven for 20 mins until well risen and golden. Cool on a wire rack for a few mins before peeling the egg and eating with the warm bread.

Bolognese

Prep: 15 mins

Cook: 40 mins

Easy

Serves 4

Ingredients

- 2 tbsp olive oil
- 2 onions , finely chopped
- 3 carrots , finely chopped
- 4 celery sticks, finely chopped
- 2 courgettes , cut into small cubes
- 4 garlic cloves , finely chopped
- 250g pack beef mince
- 1 heaped tbsp tomato purée
- 400g can chopped tomato
- 400g fettuccine
- 200g pea , frozen or fresh
- handful parsley , roughly chopped

Directions:

1. Heat the oil in large deep frying pan. Add the onions, carrots, celery, courgettes and garlic. Cook for about 10

mins or until soft, adding a few splashes of water if the mixture begins to stick. Turn up the heat and add the mince. Fry for a few mins more, breaking up the mince with the back of a spoon. Stir in tomato purée, pour over the chopped tomatoes and add a can of water. Simmer for 15 mins until the sauce is thick, then season.

2. Meanwhile, cook the fettuccine following pack instructions.

3. Tip the peas into the sauce and simmer for 2 mins more until tender. Stir through the drained pasta and parsley, then serve.

Milk chocolate pots with citrus shortbread

Prep:20 mins

Cook:30 mins plus at least 2 hrs chilling

Easy

Serves 4

Ingredients

<u>For the chocolate pots</u>
- 200g good-quality milk chocolate , chopped
- 200ml double cream
- 2 large egg yolks , lightly whisked For the shortbread
- 160g self-raising flour , plus extra for dusting
- zest 1 orange
- 110g butter , cut into cubes
- 60g golden caster sugar , plus extra for sprinkling
- 1 large egg yolk
- 100ml whipping cream

Directions:

1. Put the chocolate in a heatproof bowl. Heat the cream in a saucepan until it just boils, then pour it over the chocolate. Stir until smooth, then beat in the egg yolks. Tip the

16

mixture into a jug, then pour into four individual pots and put in the fridge to set for at least 2 hrs.

2. Meanwhile, put the flour, orange zest and butter in a large bowl and rub together until it resembles fine breadcrumbs. Add the sugar and egg yolk, mix gently and bring the biscuit dough together with your hands. Roll the shortbread out on a lightly floured surface until 1cm thick, then transfer to a baking tray lined with baking parchment. Leave to rest for 10 mins in the fridge.

3. Heat oven to 160C/140C fan/ gas 3. Bake for 23-25 mins until golden brown, then sprinkle with sugar. While still warm, cut into eight x 2cm biscuits, trimming off any excess, and leave to cool.

4. When ready to eat, whip the cream to soft peaks, then spoon on top of the chocolate pots. Serve with the shortbreads on the side.

Easy chilli con carne

Prep: 20 mins

Cook: 1 hr

Easy

Serves 4

Ingredients

2 tbsp olive oil
- 2 large onions, halved and sliced
- 3 large garlic cloves, chopped
- 2 tbsp mild chilli powder
- 2 tsp ground cumin
- 2 tsp dried oregano
- 1kg pack lean minced beef
- 400g can chopped tomato
- 2 beef stock cubes (we like Just Bouillon)
- 2 large red peppers, deseeded and cut into chunks
- 10 sundried tomatoes
- 3 x 400g cans red kidney beans, drained

Directions:

1. Heat oven to 150C/fan 130C/gas 3. Heat the oil, preferably in a large flameproof casserole, and fry the onions for 8

mins. Add the garlic, spices and oregano and cook for 1 min, then gradually add the mince, stirring well until browned. Stir in the tomatoes, add half a can of water, then crumble in the stock and season.

2. Cover and cook in the oven for 30 mins. Stir in the peppers and sundried tomatoes, then cook for 30 mins more until the peppers are tender. Stir in the beans.

3. To serve, reheat on the hob until bubbling. Serve with avocado or a big salad with avocado in it, some basmati rice or tortilla chips and a bowl of soured cream.

4. If you want to use a slow cooker, fry your onions in a pan for 8 mins, then add your garlic, spices and oregano and cook for a minute. Gradually add the mince until it's brown. Tip into your slow cooker with the tomatoes, peppers, sundried tomatoes and beans, crumble in the stock cubes and season to taste. Cook on Low for 8-10 hours, then serve as above.

Christmas to find. Rainbow fruit skewers

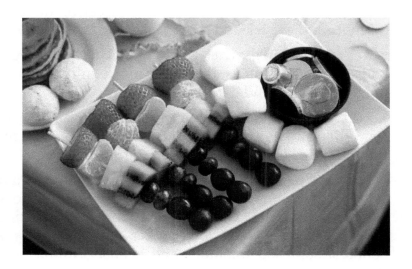

Prep:15 mins

No cook

Easy

Serves 7

Ingredients

- 7 raspberries
- 7 hulled strawberries
- 7 tangerine segments
- 7 cubes peeled mango

- 7 peeled pineapple chunks
- 7 peeled kiwi fruit chunks
- 7 green grapes
- 7 red grapes
- 14 blueberries

Directions:

Take 7 wooden skewers and thread the following fruit onto each – 1 raspberry, 1 hulled strawberry,1 tangerine segment, 1 cube of peeled mango, 1 chunk of peeled pineapple, 1 chunk of peeled kiwi,1 green and 1 red grape, and finish off with 2 blueberries. Arrange in a rainbow shape and let everyone help themselves.

Baked camembert kit

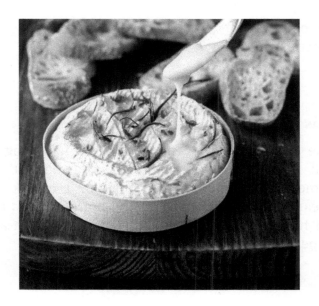

Prep:10 mins

Cook:10 mins Plus cooling

Easy

Serves 2

Ingredients
- 100g sultana
- 5 tbsp Calvados , PX Sherry, rum or brandy

- 1 boxed camembert To complete the kit
- small jar , string or ribbon and a label

Directions:

1. Heat sultanas and alcohol together until just simmering, then turn off the heat and cool completely. Spoon into a small jar and seal. Put the jar on top of the cheese and tie together with string or ribbon.

2. Keep in the fridge for up to a week until you are ready to give them away, then add a label with these instructions: 'Heat oven to 200C/fan 180C/gas 6. Unwrap the camembert, take off the wax wrapper and any other packaging. Put it back in the box but leave the lid off. Cook for 10 mins or until the centre of the cheese feels very soft. Cut a slashed cross in the centre of the cheese then tip in and over as many of the sultanas as you like. Serve with chunks of crusty bread.'

Puff pastry pizzas

Prep:20 mins

Cook:25 mins

Easy

Serves 4 (or 3 adults and 2 children)

Ingredients
- 320g sheet ready-rolled light puff pastry
- 6 tbsp tomato purée
- 1 tbsp tomato ketchup
- 1 tsp dried oregano
- 75g mozzarella or cheddar For the topping
- sweetcorn , olives, peppers, red onion, cherry tomatoes, spinach, basil

Directions:
1. Heat the oven to 200C/180C fan/gas 6. Unroll the pastry, cut into six squares and arrange over two baking trays lined with baking parchment. Use a cutlery knife to score a 1cm border around the edge of each pastry square. Bake for 15 mins, until puffed up but not cooked through.

2. While the pastry cooks, make the sauce and prepare your toppings. Mix the tomato purée, tomato ketchup, oregano

and 1 tbsp water. Grate the cheese and chop any veg or herbs you want to put on top into small pieces. Set aside.

3. Remove the pastry from the oven and squash down the middles with the back of a spoon. Divide the sauce between the pastry squares and spread it out to the puffed-up edges. Sprinkle with the cheese, then add your toppings. Bake for another 5-8 mins and serve.

Chewy cranberry choc-nut cookie kit

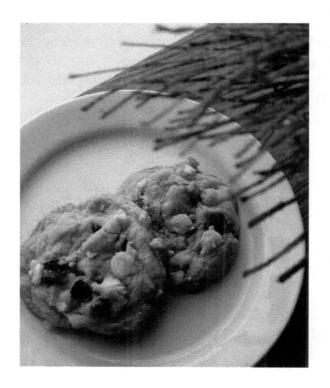

Total time: 15 mins

Ready in 15 mins

Easy

Makes 1 gift jar

Ingredients

1 large (1 litre approx) jar - Kilner or with a good screw lid
- 100g caster sugar
- 100g light muscovado sugar
- 250g self-raising flour
- 85g macadamia nut , roughly chopped
- 85g dried cranberry
- 100g white chocolate chip , buttons, or roughly chopped chunks

Directions:

Clean the jar and dry well. Layer in the Ingredients, starting with the caster sugar, followed by the muscovado, flour, nuts, cranberries and finally finishing with the white chocolate. Close the jar, then add a label with baking instructions, plus a ribbon or pretty cover if you like.

Gravadlax kit

Easy Ingredients

- 1 orange
- 1 dill plant
- small pot of black peppercorns
- 125g box of sea salt
- 500g bag of demerara sugar
- small pot of coriander seeds
- small pot of caraway seeds
- a fishmonger gift voucher (to buy a 500g boneless piece of salmon)
- pestle and mortar (optional)

Directions:

1. To use the kit: Write the following instructions on the gift tag:To make the cure for your gravadlax, zest the orange and roughly chop a large bunch of dill. Using a pestle and mortar, grind 1 /2 tbsp peppercorns, then stir in 50g sea salt, 75g sugar, 1 tsp each coriander seeds and caraway seeds, and the zest.

2. Put half the dill on a large piece of cling film and place your salmon on top. Cover with all the cure and the remaining dill, then wrap tightly. Place in a dish with something heavy on top to weigh it down.

3. Leave to cure for 24-48 hrs, turning the salmon once, then rinse well and pat dry before serving. Will keep in the fridge for up to three days.

Satay chicken & mango wraps

Prep:15 mins

Cook:15 mins

Easy

Serves 4

Ingredients

- 5 tbsp smooth peanut butter
- 160ml can coconut cream
- 1 tbsp soy sauce
- 2 tbsp mango chutney
- zest 1 lime , plus wedges to serve
- 4 skinless chicken breasts , cut into chunky pieces
- 300g pack chopped mango
- 2 carrots , grated or julienned
- handful coriander leaves (optional)
- 4 wraps , warmed

Directions:

1. In a large bowl, mix the peanut butter, coconut cream, soy, mango chutney and lime zest. Spoon half into a serving bowl and set aside. Add the chicken pieces to the large bowl and toss everything well to coat. Can be left to marinate in the fridge for up to 24 hrs.

2. Thread the chicken onto skewers (you should make 4-6), alternating the chunks with pieces of mango. Place on a baking tray lined with foil. Heat the grill to high and cook the skewers for 5 mins each side until the chicken is cooked through and starting to char on the edges. Serve in warm wraps with bowls of carrot, coriander, extra satay sauce and lime wedges for squeezing over.

Chocolate fudge Easter cakes

Cook: 15 mins

Easy

Serving 16

Ingredients

Chocolate fudge easter cakes
- 140g soft butter
- 140g golden caster sugar
- 3 medium eggs
- 100g self-raising flour
- 25g cocoa , sifted For the frosting
- 85g milk chocolate , broken
- 85g soft butter
- 140g icing sugar , sifted
- 235g/1.5oz packs white chocolate maltesers, mini foil-wrapped chocolate eggs We use Fairtrade Divine milk chocolate eggs from Waitrose

Directions:

1. Heat oven to 190C/fan 170C/gas 5 and put 16 gold cases into a fairy-cake tin. Tip all the Ingredients for the cake into a mixing bowl and beat for 2 mins with an electric hand-whisk until smooth. Divide between the cases so they

31

are two-thirds filled, then bake for 12-15 mins until risen. Cool on a wire rack.

2. For the frosting, microwave the chocolate on High for 1 min. Cream the butter and sugar together, then beat in the melted chocolate. Spread on the cakes and decorate with Maltesers and chocolate eggs.

Easter egg rocky road

Prep:25 mins

Cook:5 mins plus cooling and 1 hr chilling

Easy

Makes 8-10 bars

Ingredients

- 225g dark chocolate , broken into pieces
- 100g unsalted butter , cubed
- 2 tbsp cocoa powder
- 2 tbsp golden syrup
- 100g rich tea biscuits
- 50g mini marshmallows
- 50g dried cranberries
- 200g chocolate mini eggs

Directions:

1. Line a 20 x 30cm traybake tin with 2 sheets of cling film (in a criss-cross pattern). Put the chocolate and butter in a large bowl set over a saucepan of gently simmering water, and melt until smooth and glossy.

2. Remove from the heat and add the cocoa powder and golden syrup. Mix together until fully combined and leave to cool at room temperature for about 15 mins.

3. Put the biscuits in a freezer bag and use a rolling pin to bash them, leaving some pieces chunkier than others. Stir into the cooled chocolate with the marshmallows, cranberries and 150g of the mini eggs.

4. Pour the mix into the tin and press down with the back of a spoon until even. Scatter over the remaining mini eggs, pressing them in a little, and leave to set in the fridge for 1 hr.

5. Remove from the tin and cut into bars to serve. Will keep for up to 1 week in an airtight container.

Family meals: Mild chicken curry

Prep:10 mins

Cook:1 hr and 20 mins

Easy

Serves 2 adults, 1 child

Ingredients

- 1-1½ tsp coconut oil (we used Fushi) or sunflower oil
- 1 large onion, finely chopped
- 2 fat garlic cloves, crushed
- 1cm fresh ginger, grated or finely chopped
- 1 tsp ground coriander
- 1 tsp yellow mustard seed
- 1 tsp garam masala
- ½ tsp ground cumin
- 1 x 500g pack chicken pieces (thighs and drumsticks), or thighs
- 1 chicken stock cube
- 1 cinnamon stick
- 250g Greek yogurt, at room temperature
- 2 tbsp sultana
- handful chopped coriander, to serve (optional)

Directions:

1. Heat the oil in a heavy-based pan. Fry the onions gently for 5 – 10 mins until soft. Add the garlic, ginger, coriander, mustard seeds, garam masala and cumin and cook for 1 - 2 min allowing the aromas to release.

2. Add the chicken and cook for 10 mins over a gentle heat, flipping occasionally and making sure the spices don't catch. Pour in around 300 ml boiling water until almost covering. Stir in the stock cube and cinnamon stick. Simmer for around 45 mins - 1 hour with the lid off so there is a small amount of thickened sauce at the bottom of the pan. Remove the cinnamon stick.

3. Stir in the yogurt and sultanas, heat through gently and serve. Scatter with coriander, if using.

Simple nutty pancakes

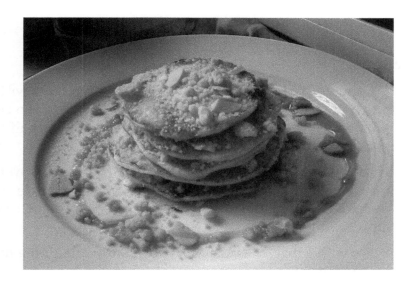

Prep: 5 mins

Cook:5 mins

Easy makes 4

Ingredients
- 150g self-raising flour
- ½ tsp baking powder
- 1 large egg
- 150ml milk
- 2 tbsp agave syrup , plus extra to serve

- 50g mixed nuts , chopped
- 2 tbsp rapeseed oil , for frying

Directions:

1. Tip the flour and baking powder into a large bowl with a pinch of salt. Make a well in the centre, then add the egg, milk and syrup. Whisk until smooth, then fold in half the nuts.

2. Heat 1 tbsp oil in a large, non-stick frying pan over a medium-high heat. Spoon two ladles of the mixture into the pan and cook for 1 min each side. Repeat to make two more.

3. Serve with a drizzle of agave syrup and the remaining nuts for extra crunch.

Flowerpot chocolate chip muffins

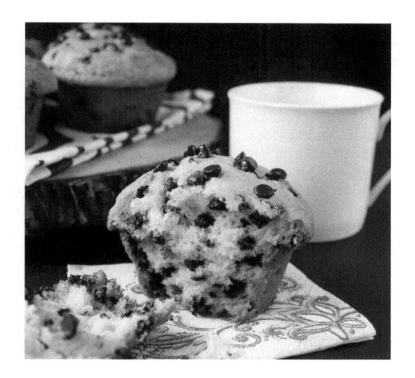

Prep: 10 mins

Cook: 12 mins - 15 mins

Easy

Makes 10 mini muffins

Ingredients

- 3 tbsp vegetable oil
- 125g plain flour
- 1 tsp baking powder
- 25g cocoa powder
- 100g golden caster sugar
- 1 large egg
- 100ml milk
- 150g milk chocolate chips
- 25g chocolate cake decorations such as vermicelli sprinkles or chocolate-coated popping candy
- 20 rice paper wafer daisies (these come in packs of 12, so get 2 packs) You will need
- 10 mini teracotta pots (see tip)

Directions:

1. Heat oven to 180C/160C fan/gas 4. Lightly oil the inside of the terracotta pots with a little vegetable oil and place on a baking tray. Place a paper mini muffin case in the bottom of each pot.

2. Put the flour, baking powder and cocoa in a bowl and stir in the sugar.

3. Crack the egg into a jug and whisk with the milk and remaining oil. Pour this over the flour and cocoa mixture, and stir in with 50g of the chocolate chips. Be careful not to overmix – you want a loose but still quite lumpy mixture. Spoon into the pots up to three-quarters full. Place in the middle of the oven and bake for 12-15 mins until risen and firm. Transfer to a wire rack (still in the pots) and leave to cool.

4. Put the rest of the chocolate chips in a small bowl and melt over a small pan of gently simmering water (don't let the

water touch the bowl), or put in a microwave-proof bowl and heat on High for 1 min until melted.

5. Spread the tops of the muffins with the melted chocolate. Sprinkle over the chocolate decorations and add 2 rice paper wafer daisies to each pot to serve. Will keep for 2 days in an airtight container.

Sticky plum flapjack bars

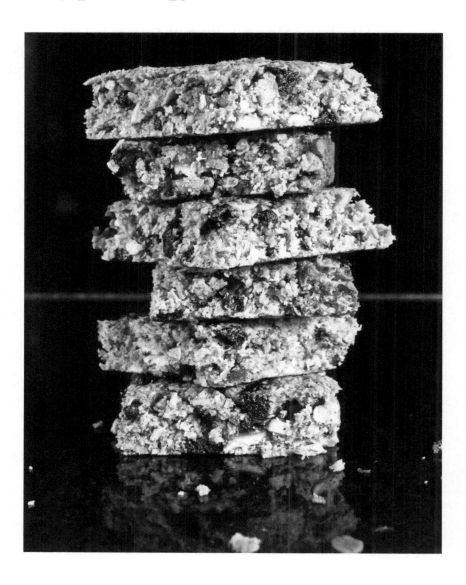

Prep:20 mins

Cook:1 hr

Easy

Makes 18

Ingredients

- 450g fresh plum , halved, stoned and roughly sliced
- ½ tsp mixed spice
- 300g light muscovado sugar
- 350g butter , plus extra for greasing
- 300g rolled porridge oats (not jumbo)
- 140g plain flour
- 50g chopped walnut pieces
- 3 tbsp golden syrup

Directions:

1. Heat oven to 200C/180C fan/gas 6. Tip the plums into a bowl. Toss with the spice, 50g of the sugar and a small pinch of salt, then set aside to macerate.

2. Gently melt the butter in a saucepan. In a large bowl, mix the oats, flour, walnut pieces and remaining sugar together, making sure there are no lumps of sugar, then stir in the butter and golden syrup until everything is combined into a loose flapjack mixture.

3. Grease a square baking tin about 20 x 20cm. Press half the oaty mix over the base of the tin, then tip over the plums and spread to make an even layer. Press the remaining oats over the plums so they are completely covered right to the sides of the tin. Bake for 45-50 mins until dark golden and starting to crisp a little around the edges. Leave to cool completely, then cut into 18 little bars. Will keep in an airtight container for 2 days or can be frozen for up to a month.

Easter chocolate bark

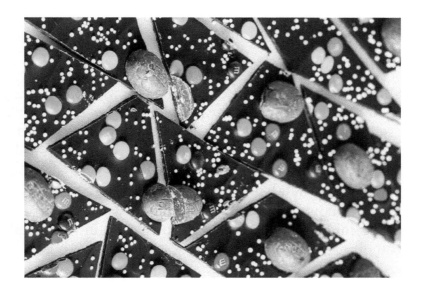

Prep: 20 mins

Cook:5 mins plus cooling

Easy

Makes enough for 6-8 gift bags

Ingredients
- 3 x 200g bars milk chocolate
- 2 x 90g packs mini chocolate eggs

• 1 heaped tsp freeze-dried raspberry pieces – or you could use crystallised petals

Directions:

1. Break the chocolate into a large heatproof bowl. Bring a pan of water to a simmer, then sit the bowl on top. The water must not touch the bottom of the bowl. Let the chocolate slowly melt, stirring now and again with a spatula. For best results, temper your chocolate (see tip).

2. Meanwhile, lightly grease then line a 23 x 33cm roasting tin or baking tray with parchment. Put three-quarters of the mini eggs into a food bag and bash them with a rolling pin until broken up a little.

3. When the chocolate is smooth, pour it into the tin. Tip the tin from side to side to let the chocolate find the corners and level out. Scatter with the smashed and whole mini eggs, followed by the freeze-dried raspberry pieces. Leave to set, then remove from the parchment and snap into shards, ready to pack in boxes or bags.

Blueberry & lemon pancakes

Prep:10 mins

Cook:20 mins

Easy Makes 14-16

Ingredients

- 200g plain flour
- 1 tsp cream of tartar
- ½ tsp bicarbonate of soda
- 1 tsp golden syrup
- 75g blueberry
- zest 1 lemon
- 200ml milk
- 1 large egg
- butter , for cooking

Directions:

1. First, put the flour, cream of tartar and bicarbonate of soda in the bowl. Mix them well with the fork. Drop the golden syrup into the dry Ingredients along with the blueberries and lemon zest.

2. Pour the milk into a measuring jug. Now break in the egg and mix well with a fork. Pour most of the milk mixture into the bowl and mix well with a rubber spatula. Keep

adding more milk until you get a smooth, thick, pouring batter.

3. Heat the frying pan and brush with a little butter. Then spoon in the batter, 1 tbsp at a time, in heaps. Bubbles will appear on top as the pancakes cook– turn them at this stage, using the metal spatula to help you. Cook until brown on the second side, then keep warm on a plate, covered with foil. Repeat until all the mixture is used up.

Chocolate fudge cupcakes

Prep:30 mins

Cook:25 mins - 30 minsPlus cooling

Easy

Makes 12

Ingredients

- 200g butter
- 200g plain chocolate , under 70% cocoa solids is fine
- 200g light, soft brown sugar
- 2 eggs , beaten
- 1 tsp vanilla extract
- 250g self-raising flour
- Smarties , sweets and sprinkles, to decorate For the icing
- 200g plain chocolate
- 100ml double cream , not fridge-cold
- 50g icing sugar

Directions:

1. Heat oven to 160C/140C fan/gas 3 and line a 12-hole muffin tin with cases. Gently melt the butter, chocolate, sugar and 100ml hot water together in a large saucepan,

49

stirring occasionally, then set aside to cool a little while you weigh the other Ingredients.

2. Stir the eggs and vanilla into the chocolate mixture. Put the flour into a large mixing bowl, then stir in the chocolate mixture until smooth. Spoon into cases until just over three-quarters full (you may have a little mixture leftover), then set aside for 5 mins before putting on a low shelf in the oven and baking for 20-22 mins. Leave to cool.

3. For the icing, melt the chocolate in a heatproof bowl over a pan of barely simmering water. Once melted, turn off the heat, stir in the double cream and sift in the icing sugar. When spreadable, top each cake with some and decorate with your favourite sprinkles and sweets.

Cheese, ham & grape kebabs

Prep: 10 mins

No cook

Easy

Serves 1

Ingredients

- 6 bocconcini (mini mozzarella balls)
- 6 grapes (a combination of red and green looks nice),
- 6 cubes of ham

Directions:

1. Using 3 short wooden skewers, thread on the mini mozzarella balls, grapes, and cubes of ham. Place in a sealable container or wrap in cling film and pop in a lunchbox. White rabbit biscuits <u>Prep</u>:1 hr and 10 mins **Cook:**45 mins

Winter warmer hearty risotto

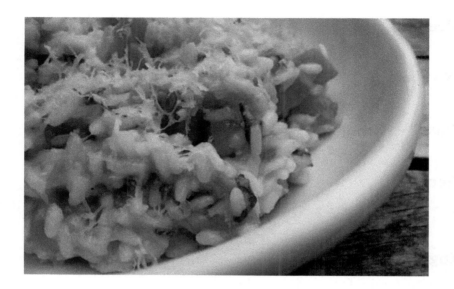

Prep:10 mins

Cook:50 mins

Easy

Serves 4

Ingredients
- 1 medium butternut squash
- 2 tbsp olive oil
- pinch of nutmeg , or pinch of cinnamon

- 1 red onion , finely chopped
- 1 vegetable stock cube
- 2 garlic cloves , crushed
- 500g risotto rice (we used arborio)
- 100g frozen peas
- 320g sweetcorn , drained
- 2 tbsp grated parmesan (or vegetarian alternative)
- handful chopped mixed herbs of your choice

Directions:

1. Heat oven to 200C/180C fan/gas 6. Peel the butternut squash, slice it in half, then scoop out and discard the seeds.2 Cut the flesh of the butternut squash into small cubes and put in a mixing bowl.

2. Drizzle 1 tbsp olive oil over the squash, and season with black pepper, and nutmeg or cinnamon. Transfer the squash to a roasting tin and roast in the oven for about 25 mins until cooked through, then set aside.

3. Heat the remaining oil in a large saucepan over a low heat. Add the onion and cover the pan with a tight-fitting lid. Allow the onion to cook without colouring for 5-10 mins, stirring occasionally.

4. In a measuring jug, make up 1.5 litres of stock from boiling water and the stock cube. Stir well until the stock cube has dissolved. When the onion is soft, remove the lid and add the garlic to the onion pan. Leave it to cook for 1 min more.

5. Rinse the rice under cold water. Turn up the heat on the pan and add the rice to the onion and garlic, stirring well for 1 min. Pour a little of the hot stock into the pan and stir in until the liquid is absorbed by the rice.

6. Gradually add the rest of the stock to the pan, a little at a time, stirring constantly, waiting until each addition of stock is absorbed before adding more. Do this until the rice is cooked through and creamy – you may not need all the stock. This should take 15-20 mins. Take the roasting tin out of the oven – the squash should be soft and cooked.

7. Add the squash, peas and sweetcorn to the risotto and gently stir it in. Season to taste. Take the risotto pan off the heat and stir in the Parmesan and herbs. Put the lid back on the pan and let the risotto stand for 2-3 mins before serving.

Prawn & mango salad

Prep:10 mins

No cook

Easy

Serves 2

Ingredients

- ½ avocado , peeled and cut into cubes, see tip, below left
- squeeze of lemon juice
- 50g small cooked prawns
- 1 mango cheek, peeled and cut into cubes
- 4 cherry tomatoes , halved
- finger-sized piece cucumber , chopped
- handful baby spinach leaves
- couple of mint leaves , very finely shredded
- 1-2 tsp sweet chilli sauce

Directions:

Mix the avocado with the lemon juice, then toss with the prawns, mango, tomatoes, cucumber, spinach and mint. Pack into a lunchbox and drizzle over the sweet chilli sauce, then chill until ready to eat.

Marshmallows dipped in chocolate

Prep: 10 mins

Cook:5 mins Plus setting time

Easy

Makes 26 approx

Ingredients

- 50g white chocolate
- 50g milk chocolate
- selection of cake sprinkles
- 1 bag marshmallows (about 200g)
- 1 pack lollipop sticks

Directions:

1. Heat the chocolate in separate bowls over simmering water or on a low setting in the microwave. Allow to cool a little.

2. Put your chosen sprinkles on separate plates. Push a cake pop or lolly stick into a marshmallow about half way in. Dip into the white or milk chocolate, allow the excess to drip off then dip into the sprinkles of your choice. Put into a tall glass to set. Repeat with each marshmallow.

Bacon Bolognese

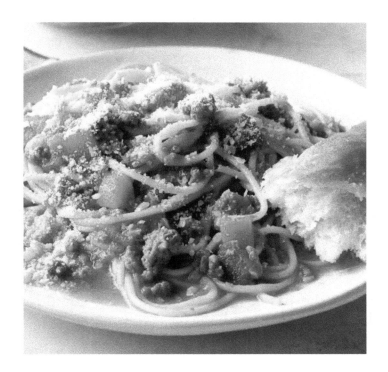

Prep: 10 mins

Cook: 12 mins

Easy

Serves 4

Ingredients

- 400g spaghetti
- 1 tsp olive oil
- 2 large carrots , finely diced
- 3 celery sticks, finely diced
- 200g pack smoked bacon lardon
- 190g jar sundried tomato pesto
- 8-12 basil leaves , shredded (optional)

Directions:

1. Boil the spaghetti following pack instructions. Meanwhile, heat the oil in a non-stick pan. Add the carrots, celery and bacon, and stir well. Cover the pan and cook, stirring occasionally, for 10 mins until the veg has softened.

2. Tip in the pesto, warm through, then stir through the drained spaghetti with the basil, if using.

Vanilla chick biscuit pops

Prep: 15 mins

Cook: 6 mins - 7 mins plus chilling and cooling

Easy Makes 15-18 biscuits

Ingredients

- 200g unsalted butter , at room temperature
- 100g golden caster sugar
- 1 medium egg , beaten
- 1 tsp vanilla extract
- 200g plain flour , plus extra for dusting
- 200g icing sugar
- 2 tbsp milk
- few drops yellow food colouring
- 75g unsweetened desiccated coconut
- 50g small chocolate chips
- 25g orange or white fondant icing , plus a few drops orange food colouring You will need
- 15-18 lolly sticks (see tip)
- ribbon , to decorate (optional)

Directions:

1. Put half the butter and all the sugar in a bowl. Using an electric whisk or wooden spoon, beat together until

smooth and creamy. Beat in the egg and half the vanilla extract until thoroughly combined.

2. Tip the flour into the mixture and mix on a low speed until it comes together to form a dough. Gather up into a ball, wrap in cling film and chill in the fridge for 20 mins.

3. Heat oven to 180C/160C fan/gas 4. Line 2 baking trays with baking parchment. Put the biscuit dough on a lightly floured surface and roll out until about 5mm thick. Cut out the biscuits using a 6cm round cutter. Transfer the biscuits to the prepared trays and insert the lolly sticks into the sides, just a quarter of the way through. Bake for 6-7 mins until the edges are golden brown, then carefully transfer to a wire rack and allow to cool completely before decorating.

4. Meanwhile, make some buttercream frosting. Place the remaining softened butter in a bowl and beat with a wooden spoon. Slowly add the icing sugar, 1 tbsp at a time, until thoroughly incorporated and you have a smooth, creamy mixture. Add a little milk and the remaining vanilla extract with a few drops of food colouring to give a pale yellow colour. Chill for 5 mins.

5. Put the desiccated coconut in a small bowl, add a few drops of yellow food colouring and mix well until the coconut is coloured pale yellow.

6. Spread the buttercream frosting over one side of the biscuit and sprinkle with the coconut. Add 2 chocolate chip eyes to each. Pinch a little orange fondant icing and shape into a beak and press into the mixture. Decorate with a ribbon, if you like, and serve. Will keep for 2 days in an airtight container.

Christmas pudding Rice Krispie cakes

Prep: 30 hrs

Cook:5 mins plus chilling

Easy

Makes 10 - 12

Ingredients

• 50g rice pops (we used Rice Krispies)
• 30g raisin , chopped
• 50g butter
• 100g milk chocolate , broken into pieces
• 2 tbsp crunchy peanut butter
• 30g mini marshmallow
• 80g white chocolate
• ready-made icing holly leaves (we used Sainsbury's Christmas cake decorations)

Directions:

1. Put the rice pops and raisins into a bowl. Put the butter, milk chocolate, peanut butter and marshmallows into a small saucepan. Place on a medium to low heat and stir until the chocolate and butter have melted but the marshmallows are just beginning to melt.

2. Pour onto the rice pops and stir until well coated. Line an egg cup with cling film. Press about a tablespoon of the mixture into the egg cup. Press firmly and then remove, peel off the cling film and place the pudding into a cake case, flat-side down. Repeat with the remaining mixture. Chill until firm.

3. Melt the white chocolate in the microwave or in bowl over a saucepan of barely simmering water. Spoon a little chocolate over the top of each pudding. Top with icing holly leaves.

Yummy chocolate log

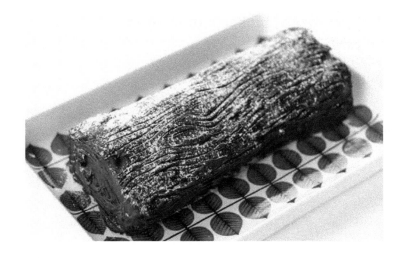

Prep:30 mins

Cook:10 mins

More effort

Serves 8

Ingredients

For the cake
• 3 eggs
• 85g golden caster sugar
• 85g plain flour (minus 2 tbsp)

- 2 tbsp cocoa powder
- ½ tsp baking powder For the filling & icing
- 50g butter, plus extra for the tin
- 140g dark chocolate , broken into squares
- 1 tbsp golden syrup
- 284ml pot double cream
- 200g icing sugar, sifted
- 2-3 extra strong mints, crushed (optional)
- icing sugar and holly sprigs to decorate - ensure you remove the berries before serving

Directions:

1. Heat the oven to 200C/180C fan/gas 6. Butter and line a 23 x 32cm Swiss roll tin with baking parchment. Beat the eggs and golden caster sugar together with an electric whisk for about 8 mins until thick and creamy.

2. Mix the flour, cocoa powder and baking powder together, then sift onto the egg mixture. Fold in very carefully, then pour into the tin. Tip the tin from side to side to spread the mixture into the corners. Bake for 10 mins.

3. Lay a sheet of baking parchment on a work surface. When the cake is ready, tip it onto the parchment, peel off the lining paper, then roll the cake up from its longest edge with the paper inside. Leave to cool.

4. To make the icing, melt the butter and dark chocolate together in a bowl over a pan of hot water. Take from the heat and stir in the golden syrup and 5 tbsp double cream. Beat in the icing sugar until smooth.

5. Whisk the remaining double cream until it holds its shape. Unravel the cake, spread the cream over the top, scatter

over the crushed extra strong mints, if using, then carefully roll up again into a log.

6. Cut a thick diagonal slice from one end of the log. Lift the log on to a plate, then arrange the slice on the side with the diagonal cut against the cake to make a branch. Spread the icing over the log and branch (don't cover the ends), then use a fork to mark the icing to give the effect of tree bark. Scatter with unsifted icing sugar to resemble snow, and decorate with holly.

Easy Easter nests

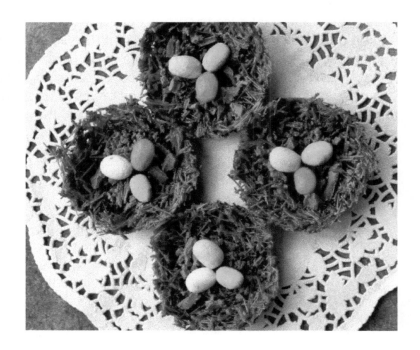

Prep: 25 mins

Cook:8 mins Plus chilling

Easy

Makes 12

Ingredients

- 200g milk chocolate , broken into pieces
- 85g shredded wheat , crushed
- 2 x 100g bags mini chocolate eggs You'll also need
- cupcake cases

Directions:

1. Melt the chocolate in a small bowl placed over a pan of barely simmering water. Pour the chocolate over the shredded wheat and stir well to combine.

2. Spoon the chocolate wheat into 12 cupcake cases and press the back of a teaspoon in the centre to create a nest shape. Place 3 mini chocolate eggs on top of each nest. Chill the nests in the fridge for 2 hrs until set.

No-fuss fish pie

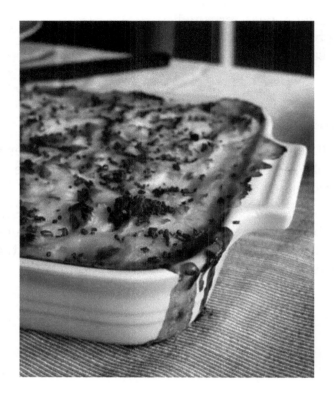

Prep:30 mins

Cook:25 mins

Easy

Serves 4

Ingredients

- 400ml milk
- 1 bay leaf
- 1 garlic clove , finely chopped
- 1 medium onion , thinly sliced
- 300g skinless, boneless fish (we used a mix of salmon, smoked haddock and cod)
- 5 medium potatoes
- 3 parsnips , peeled
- 2 eggs
- 125g (drained weight) can sweetcorn
- 125g frozen peas
- 2 tbsp mixed chopped herbs (lemon thyme, coriander and chives are nice)
- zest 0.5 lemon
- small pack of cooked small prawns (optional)
- 4 tsp crème fraîche
- pinch of ground nutmeg
- pinch of white pepper
- 1 tsp wholegrain mustard
- 25g butter
- 50g grated cheese
- steamed carrots , to serve
- steamed broccoli , to serve

Directions:

1. Heat oven to 190C/170C fan/gas 5. Put the milk in a saucepan with the bay leaf, garlic and onion. Add the fish and poach on a medium heat for 15 mins. The milk should be just covering the fish, if not, add a little more.

2. Cut the potatoes and parsnips into equal-sized pieces and put in a saucepan. Cover with cold water and a lid, bring to the boil, then simmer on a medium heat for 10 mins, or until the potatoes and parsnips are soft (not falling apart).

69

3. Meanwhile, gently put the eggs in a small pan of water and bring to the boil. Cook for 7 mins, then transfer to a bowl of cold water and leave to cool. Once cool, peel and chop them.

4. When the fish is cooked (it should be firm to the touch and flake easily), remove from the milk, along with the onion, using a slotted spoon. Strain the milk into a jug and keep it for the mash.

5. Flake the fish into bite-sized chunks (checking for bones) and place in the bottom of a casserole dish, then add the onion, sweetcorn and peas.

6. Add the herbs, lemon zest, prawns (if using), hard-boiled eggs and the crème fraîche. Season and mix well.

7. Drain the parsnips and potatoes in a colander, and return to the saucepan. Add the nutmeg, white pepper, mustard and a knob of butter and mash well

8. Taste to check the seasoning. Cover the fish filling with the mashed potato and, using a fork, create a wavy pattern, if you like. Sprinkle over the grated cheese.

9. Place in the oven for 20 mins or until the cheese is melted and golden brown, remove from the oven using oven gloves and serve with steamed crunchy carrots and broccoli.

Carrot cake traybake

Prep:30 mins

Cook:30 mins Plus cooling

Easy

Makes 6-12

Ingredients

- 200g carrots , peeled
- 175g soft brown sugar
- 200g self-raising flour
- 1 tsp bicarbonate of soda
- 2 tsp cinnamon
- zest 1 orange
- 2 eggs
- 150ml sunflower oil For the icing
- 50g softened butter
- 75g icing sugar
- 200g soft cheese
- sprinkles (optional)

Directions:

1. Line an 18cm square tin with baking parchment. Ask your grown-up helper to turn the oven on to 180C/160C fan/gas 2. Grate the carrots on the fine side of the grater, then tip them into a large bowl.

2. Sift the sugar, flour, bicarb and cinnamon on top of the carrot, then add the orange zest and mix everything around a bit.

3. Break the eggs into a bowl (scoop out any bits of shell), then add them to the bowl along with the oil. Mix everything together well

4. Scoop the cake mix into your tin and level the top. Ask a grown-up to put it in the oven for 30 minutes or until the cake is cooked. Cool.

5. To make the icing, mix the butter and icing sugar together, then stir in the soft cheese until smooth.

6. When the cake is cool, spread the top with the icing and cut into squares. Decorate with sprinkles, if you like.

Choco-dipped tangerines

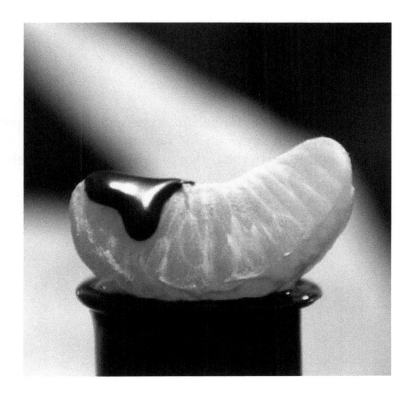

Prep: 10 mins

Easy

Serves 1

Ingredients

- 1 tangerine , peeled and segmented
- 10g dark chocolate , melted

Directions:

Dip half of each tangerine segment in the melted chocolate, then put on a baking sheet lined with parchment. Keep in the fridge for 1 hr to set completely, or overnight if you prefer.

Chocolate crunch bars

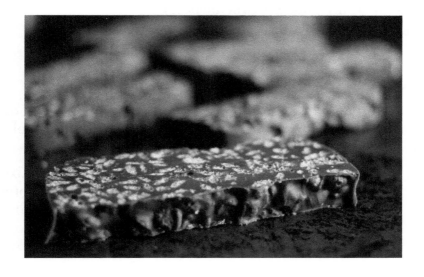

Prep: 20 mins plus chilling

Cook: 5 mins

Easy

Cuts into 12

Ingredients

- 100g butter , roughly chopped
- 300g dark chocolate (such as Bournville), broken into squares
- 3 tbsp golden syrup
- 140g rich tea biscuit , roughly crushed

- 12 pink marshmallows , quartered (use scissors)
- 2 x 55g bars Turkish delight , halved and sliced (or use Maltesers, Milky Way or Crunchie bars)

Directions:

1. Gently melt the butter, chocolate and syrup in a pan over a low heat, stirring frequently until smooth, then cool for about 10 mins.

2. Stir the biscuits and sweets into the pan until well mixed, then pour into a 17cm square tin lined with foil and spread the mixture to roughly level it. Chill until hard, then cut into fingers.

Fruity Neapolitan lolly loaf

Prep: 25 mins 25 mins plus 8 hours freezing time

Easy

Serves 8

Ingredients
- 200g peaches nectarines or apricots (or a mixture), stoned
- 200g strawberries or raspberries (or a mixture), hulled
- 450ml double cream
- ½ x 397g can condensed milk
- 2 tsp vanilla extract
- orange and pink food colouring (optional)
- 8 wooden lolly sticks

Directions:

1. Put the peaches, nectarines or apricots in a food processor and pulse until they're chopped and juicy but still with some texture. Scrape into a bowl. Repeat with the berries and scrape into another bowl.

2. Pour the cream, condensed milk and vanilla into a third bowl and whip until just holding soft peaks. Add roughly a third of the mixture to the peaches and another third to the berries, and mix both until well combined. Add a drop of orange food colouring to the peach mixture and a drop of pink food colouring to the berry mixture if you want a

77

really vibrant colour. Line a 900g loaf tin or terrine mould with cling film (look for a long thin one, ours was 23 x 7 x 8cm), then pour in the berry mixture. Freeze for 2 hrs and chill the remaining mixtures in the fridge.

3. Once the bottom layer is frozen, remove the vanilla mixture from the fridge and pour over the berry layer. The bottom layer should now be firm enough to support your lolly sticks, so place these, evenly spaced, along the length of the loaf tin, pushing down gently until they stand up straight. Return to the freezer for another 2 hrs.

4. Once the vanilla layer is frozen, pour over the peach mixture, easing it around the lolly sticks. Return to the freezer for a further 4 hrs or until completely frozen. Remove from the freezer 10 mins before serving. Use the cling film to help you remove the loaf from the tin. Take to the table on a board and slice off individual lollies for your guests. Any leftovers can be kept in the freezer for up to 2 weeks.

Crisp chicken bites

Prep: 10 mins

Cook: 15 mins

Easy

Serve 12 for lunch

Ingredients
- 4 boneless chicken breast fillets
- 6 tbsp red pesto
- 3 large handfuls breadcrumbs , frsh or dried (about 300g/10oz)
- olive oil

Directions:
1. Cut the chicken breasts into small chunks, each about the size of a marble (you should get roughly 15 pieces per breast). Put the pesto in a bowl and mix together with the chicken until coated all over. Tip the breadcrumbs into a large freezer bag.

2. Add the chicken pieces in batches to the bag and give it a good shake to coat. Place a piece of greaseproof paper on a baking sheet, then lay the chicken pieces on the sheet, making sure none of them are touching. Put in the freezer

and, when frozen solid, take off the baking sheet and store in a container or freezer bag.

3. To cook, heat oven to 220C/fan 200C/ gas 7. Pour a little oil onto a shallow baking tray, just enough to cover it. Put the tray in the oven and let it heat up for 5 mins. Tip the chicken onto the sheet and return to the oven for 10-15 mins until crisp and cooked through.

Stuffed jacket potatoes

Prep:20 mins

Cook:1 hr and 15 mins

Easy

Ingredients

- 4 medium potatoes
- 100g strong cheddar, grated, plus extra for topping
- 100g sweetcorn
- 100g mixed pepper, diced
- small handful fresh herbs, such as oregano, basil, coriander, dill or thyme

Directions:

1. Equipment you will need: medium mixing bowl, small mixing bowl, dessertspoon, fork, baking tray, grater, oven gloves.

2. Get an adult to heat the oven to 200C/180C fan/gas 6 and bake the potatoes for about 1 hr until cooked and the skins are crispy. Leave to cool completely. This can be done up to 2 days ahead.

3. To stuff the jacket potatoes, heat the oven to 200C/180C fan/gas 6. Ask an adult to cut the potatoes in half. Using a spoon, carefully scoop out the middle of the potato, leaving

the skin unbroken (like a boat). Place the scooped potato into a mixing bowl.

4. Using the fork, mash the potato until there are no lumps. Add the cheese, sweetcorn and peppers and mix well. Gently pick the leaves from the herbs. You can rip the larger leaves into smaller pieces. Stir the herbs into the cheesy potato mixture.

5. Using the spoon, carefully scoop the mixture back into the potato boats. Make sure that you use all the mixture up. Sprinkle with a little extra grated cheese and place on a baking tray. Using oven gloves, place the tray in the oven and bake for 10-15 mins until golden.

Millionaire's chocolate tart

Prep:30 mins

Cook:55 mins Plus chilling

More effort

Serves 10

Ingredients

- 375g pack dessert shortcrust pastry
- 1 tsp vanilla paste or extract
- flour , for dusting
- 250g/9oz caramel (we used Carnation caramel from a can)
- 100g 70% plain chocolate , broken into pieces
- 100g white chocolate , broken into pieces
- 6 tbsp melted butter
- 2 eggs , plus 3 egg yolks
- 4 tbsp golden caster sugar
- icing sugar and single cream, to serve (optional)

Directions:

1. Break the pastry into chunks and drop into a food processor. Drizzle over the vanilla paste and pulse until the vanilla is speckled through the pastry (the extract should be completely absorbed). Tip out onto a floured surface, bring together into a ball, then roll out to line a 23cm tart

tin (leave any overhanging pastry as you will trim this away when the tart is baked). Chill for 30 mins.

2. Heat oven to 200C/180C fan/gas 6. Line the pastry with greaseproof paper. Fill with baking beans, bake blind for 15-20 mins, then remove the paper and beans and bake for 5-10 mins more until pale golden. Carefully spread caramel over the base and set aside while you make the filling. Lower oven to 180C/160C fan/gas 4.

3. Melt the chocolates in a bowl over a pan of barely simmering water, then stir in the melted butter. Whisk the eggs, yolks and sugar together with an electric whisk in a large mixing bowl for 10 mins, until pale and thick enough to leave a trail when the beaters are lifted up. Fold in the melted chocolate with a large metal spoon, then scrape into the tin.

4. Bake for 20-25 mins – the surface should be set and puffed but still with a slight wobble. Cool, then chill for at least 3 hrs or overnight, before dusting with icing sugar and serving.

Eyeball & hand fruit punch

Prep:10 mins plus overnight freezing

No cook

Easy

Serves 14-15

Ingredients

- 425g can lychees
- 225g jar cocktail cherries
- 15 raisins
- 1 litre carton blueberry, blackberry or purple grape juice , chilled
- 1 litre carton cherry or cranberry juice , chilled
- 1litre sparkling water , chilled You'll also need
- 2 pairs powder-free disposable gloves

Directions:

1. Rinse the disposable gloves and fill each with water. Tie a knot in the top of each as you would a balloon, or use a tight bag clip to hold the opening closed. Freeze overnight.

2. Drain the lychees and cocktail cherries, reserving the juices in a jug. Push a raisin into one end of each cherry, then push the cherries into the lychees to make 'eyeballs'.

85

3. Tip all of the juices, plus the reserved lychee and cherry juices, into a large bowl with the 'eyeballs'. Carefully peel the gloves from the ice hands, add to the punch, then top up with the sparkling water.

Rudolph cupcakes

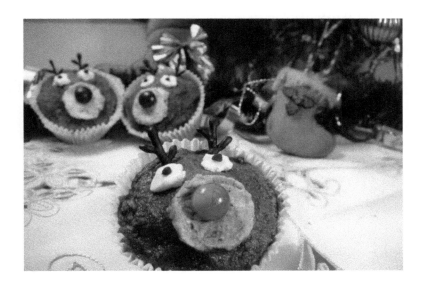

Prep:35 mins

Cook:30 mins Plus cooling

Easy

Makes 12

Ingredients
- 200g butter , cubed
- 200g plain chocolate , broken into squares
- 200g light soft brown sugar

- 2 large eggs , beaten
- 1 tsp vanilla extract
- 250g self-raising flour For the icing
- 200g plain chocolate , broken into squares
- 100ml double cream , not fridge-cold
- 50g icing sugar For the reindeers
- 12 large milk chocolate buttons (we used Cadbury Dairy Milk Giant Buttons)
- 24 white chocolate buttons
- 12 red Smarties
- black icing pens
- mini pretzels , carefully cut in half horizontally

Directions:

1. Get started: Heat oven to 160C/140C fan/gas 3. Line a 12-hole muffin tin with paper cases. Gently melt the butter, chocolate, sugar and 100ml hot water together in a large saucepan, stirring occasionally. Set aside to cool a little while you weigh the other Ingredients.

2. Make your cakes: Stir the eggs and vanilla into the chocolate mixture. Put the flour in a large mixing bowl, and stir in the chocolate mixture until smooth. Spoon into the cases until just over three-quarters full. Bake on a low shelf in the oven for 20-22 mins. Leave to cool.

3. Ice the tops: To make the icing, melt the chocolate in a heatproof bowl over a pan of barely simmering water. Once melted, turn off the heat, stir in the double cream, sift in the icing sugar and mix well. When spreadable, top each cake with some icing.

4. Have fun decorating: Position a milk chocolate button on top of each cake, then 2 white chocolate buttons above it.

Use a little icing as glue to stick a red Smartie onto the milk chocolate button for a nose. Then use your icing pens to draw black dots on the white buttons for eyes. Stick 2 pretzel top halves into the top of each cake for antlers, and stick the bottom half of a pretzel under the Smartie for a mouth. These cakes will keep in a sealed container for up to 3 days, but we doubt they'll last that long!

Stripy hummus salad jars

Prep: 15 mins

No cook

Easy

6 jars

Ingredients

- 140g frozen soya beans or peas
- 200g tub hummus (reserve 2 tbsp for the dressing)
- 2 red peppers (or a mixture of colours) finely chopped
- Half cucumber , finely chopped
- 200g cherry tomatoes , quartered
- 2 large carrots
- small pack basil
- 2 large carrots , peeled and grated
- 4 tbsp pumpkin seeds (optional) For the dressing
- zest and juice 1 lemon
- 1 tbsp clear honey
- 2 tbsp hummus (from the tub, above)

Directions:

1. First make the dressing. Put the Ingredients in a jam jar with 1 tbsp water. Screw on the lid and shake well. Set aside.

2. Bring a small pan of water to the boil, add the beans or peas and cook for 1 min until tender. Drain and run under cold water until cool. Divide the remaining hummus between 6 large jam jars. Top with the drained soya beans or peas, peppers, cucumber, tomatoes, basil leaves, carrots and pumpkin seeds, if using. Screw on the lids and chill until needed. Will keep in the fridge for 24 hrs.

3. When ready to serve, pass around the jars and let everyone pour over a little dressing.

Toffee popcorn bark

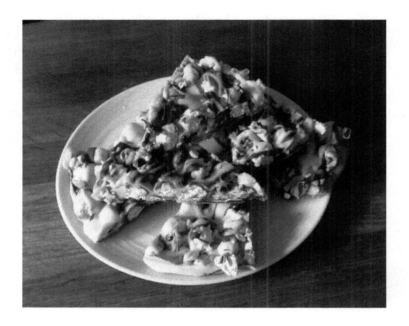

Prep:10 mins

Cook:5 mins

Easy

Serves 8

Ingredients

- 200g milk chocolate
- 200g white chocolate
- x bags toffee popcorn

Directions:

1. Line a 20 x 30cm baking tray with baking parchment. Melt the milk chocolate and white chocolate separately, then allow to cool slightly.

2. Pour most of the chocolate onto the tray, roughly swirling together. Sprinkle over the toffee popcorn, then drizzle over the remaining milk and white chocolate, and chill until set. Break into big chunks before serving.

Rigatoni sausage bake

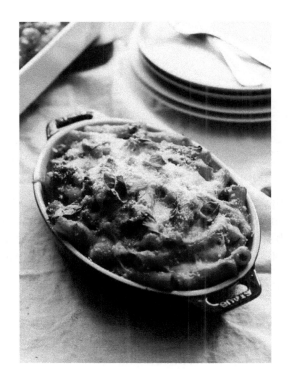

Prep: 20 mins

Cook: 45 mins - 50 mins

More effort

Serves 6

Ingredients

- 400g good quality pork sausage
- 1 tbsp olive oil
- 1 onion, chopped
- 1 large carrot, grated
- 150ml red wine
- 300ml vegetable stock
- 3 tbsp tomato purée For the sauce
- 50g butter
- 50g plain flour
- 600ml milk
- freshly grated nutmeg
- 500g rigatoni or penne
- 200g fresh spinach
- 140g mature cheddar, grated

Directions:

1. Slit the sausages and remove them from their skins, then chop them into small pieces. Heat the oil in a pan, add the onion and fry for 5 minutes, until softened and lightly browned. Stir in the sausages and fry until lightly coloured. Add the carrot, then stir in the wine, stock, tomato purée, and season.

2. Bring to the boil, then simmer uncovered for about 15 minutes until thickened. Taste and season. Set aside.

3. Put the butter, flour and milk in a pan. Gently heat, whisking, until thickened and smooth. Add a sprinkle of freshly grated nutmeg, season, then simmer for 2 minutes.

4. Preheat the oven to 190C/Gas 5/fan 170C. Bring a large pan of salted water to the boil. Add the pasta, stir well, then

cook, uncovered, for 10-12 minutes, until tender. Remove from the heat, stir in the spinach and, when just wilted, drain well.

5. Tip half the pasta into a shallow ovenproof dish, about 2.2 litre/4 pint, and level. Spoon over the sausage sauce, then cover with the remaining pasta. Pour the white sauce evenly over the top and sprinkle with the cheddar. Bake for 20-25 minutes until golden brown. Leave for 5 minutes before serving.

Shimmering forest cake

Prep: 30 mins Plus drying

Easy

Ingredients

To cover the cake
- 20cm/8inch round fruitcake
- 3 tbsp apricot jam , warmed
- icing sugar , for dusting
- 750g natural-coloured marzipan
- 750g white ready-to-roll icing To decorate
- 500g white ready-to-roll icing
- green food colouring paste
- 200g icing sugar , plus extra for dusting
- 2Christmas tree cutters , about 5cm and 10cm tall
- 1 egg white
- edible sparkles , available from cookshops
- green Smarties and silver chocolate buttons (optional)

Directions:

1. Cover the cake with marzipan and white icing. (See 5 for more information).

2. Knead the ready-to-roll icing, then split into three balls. Leave one ball white, and knead a little green colouring into the other two to give two different shades of green. Roll out each ball to about 5mm thick on a work surface lightly dusted with icing sugar. Stamp out about 15 tree

shapes using tree cutters, then leave to dry for a few hours or overnight.

3. Once firm, lift half of the trees onto a cooling rack. Combine the 200g icing sugar and egg white to make an icing, then drizzle it over the trees with a teaspoon. Scatter with edible sparkles and leave to dry again until solid.

4. Put a little icing on the back of each tree and press the trees around the edge of the cake, overlapping some to give a 3-D effect. Scatter the sweets over the top of the cake to finish. Can be iced up to a week ahead.

5. To cover a cake with marzipan, first brush the cake all over with a thin layer of warmed apricot jam. Dust the work surface with icing sugar, then roll out the marzipan evenly until you have a 5mm1cm thick round, about 40cm across for a 20cm cake. Lift over the cake, using a rolling pin to help, then smooth with your hands and trim off the excess. Leave to dry overnight or for a few hours. Lightly brush the marzipan all over with cooled, boiled water. Roll the icing out as you did the marzipan, then smooth with your hands, trim off the excess and leave to dry.

Asian chicken salad

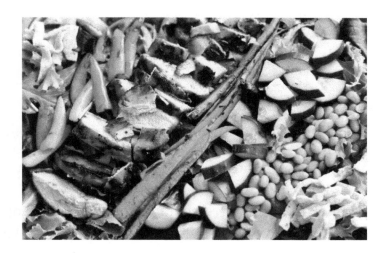

Prep:10 mins

Cook:10 mins

Easy

Serves 2

Ingredients

- 1 boneless, skinless chicken breast
- 1 tbsp fish sauce
- zest and juice ½ lime (about 1 tbsp)
- 1 tsp caster sugar
- 100g bag mixed salad leaves

- large handful coriander , roughly chopped
- ¼ red onion , thinly sliced
- ½ chilli , deseeded and thinly sliced
- ¼ cucumber , halved lengthways, sliced

Directions:

1. Cover the chicken with cold water, bring to the boil, then cook for 10 mins. Remove from the pan and tear into shreds. Stir together the fish sauce, lime zest, juice and sugar until sugar dissolves.

2. Place the leaves and coriander in a container, then top with the chicken, onion, chilli and cucumber. Place the dressing in a separate container and toss through the salad when ready to eat.

Cheeseburgers

Prep:15 mins

Cook:20 mins

Makes 12

Ingredients

- 1kg minced beef
- 300g breadcrumbs
- 140g extra-mature or mature cheddar , grated
- 4 tbsp Worcestershire sauce
- 1 small bunch parsley , finely chopped
- 2 eggs , beaten To serve
- split burger buns
- sliced tomatoes
- red onion slices
- lettuce , tomato sauce, coleslaw, wedges or fries

Directions:

1. Crumble the mince in a large bowl, then tip in the breadcrumbs, cheese, Worcestershire sauce, parsley and eggs with 1 tsp ground pepper and 1-2 tsp salt. Mix with your hands to combine everything thoroughly.

2. Shape the mix into 12 burgers. Chill until ready to cook for up to 24 hrs. Or freeze for up to 3 months. Just stack between squares of baking parchment to stop the burgers

101

sticking together, then wrap well. Defrost overnight in the fridge before cooking.

3. To cook the burgers, heat grill to high. Grill burgers for 6-8 mins on each side until cooked through. Meanwhile, warm as many buns as you need in a foil-covered tray below the grilling burgers. Let everyone assemble their own, served with their favourite accompaniments.

Fish cake fingers

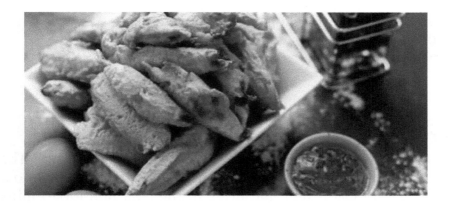

Prep: 30 mins

Cook: 40 mins

Easy

Makes 8

Ingredients
- 800g floury potato
- 2 skinless salmon fillets (about 250g), cut into chunks
- 3 smoked mackerel fillets (about 140g)
- zest 1 lemon , saving juice to serve
- plain flour , for dusting
- 3 eggs
- 100g dried breadcrumb

- 3 tbsp sunflower oil , plus more if needed To serve
- 6 tbsp mayonnaise
- lemon juice , from above
- 1 small garlic clove , chopped (optional)
- 200g frozen pea , cooked
- few handfuls watercress

Directions:

1. <u>KIDS</u>: The writing in bold is for you <u>GROWN-UPS</u>: The rest is for you. Make some mash. Tip the potatoes into a pan of cold water and bring to the boil. Boil for 10 mins then lower the heat and drop in the salmon. Turn down the heat and simmer for about 3-5 mins more until the fish is cooked. Lift the fish onto a plate with a slotted spoon. Continue cooking the potatoes until soft, then drain. Tip the potatoes into a bowl and get your child to mash them.

2. Flake the fish. While the potatoes cook, peel away the skin from the mackerel fillets and get your child to flake the meat into a small bowl – they can taste some at this point, if they like.

3. Mix it all up. Add the lemon zest to the potato, and mash some more. Then add all the flaked fish and mix together well – don't worry about breaking up the fish. If you want, divide the mix in half and add any grown-up Ingredients at this stage. Leave until cool enough to handle.

4. Roll out into long sausages. Lightly flour a surface and crack the eggs into a dish. Get your child to whisk them while you tip the breadcrumbs into another dish. Then ask them to divide the mash into eight and roll them on the flour into long, fat cylinders.

5. Dip them in egg. Working methodically, roll the sausages carefully in the egg.

6. Coat in crunchy breadcrumbs. Once the sausages are completely coated in egg, roll them in the Once the sausages are completely coated in egg, roll them in the 3 days, or frozen for 1 month. To cook from frozen, Heat oven to 180C/160C fan/gas 4. Drizzle some olive oil over the Fish cake fingers and bake for 25-30 mins, until cooked through and golden.

7. Get a grown-up to cook them. Heat the oil in a frying pan and cook the fingers in batches. Sizzle them for 8-10 mins, turning regularly until completely golden, then lift them out onto kitchen paper to drain. Keep them warm in a low oven while you cook the rest.

8. Make a tasty sauce. While you are cooking the fingers, your child can mix the mayonnaise with the lemon juice and garlic – then get them to tip it into a small dish. Serve the fish cake fingers on a plate with the peas, watercress and some of the mayonnaise dip on the side.

Cauliflower cheese pasta bake

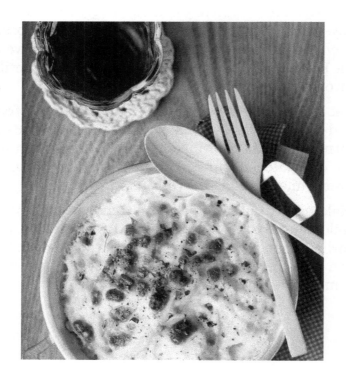

Prep: 20 mins

Cook: 1 hr

Easy

Serves 4

Ingredients

- 1 cauliflower, broken down into florets, core sliced, leaves removed and reserved, thick stems sliced
- 2 tbsp olive oil
- 6 shallots , sliced
- 1 tsp caster sugar
- 1 thyme sprig
- 2 tbsp white wine
- 100g large pasta shapes, such as conchiglioni
- 20g butter
- 1 bay leaf
- 2 tbsp plain flour
- 600ml milk
- 100g mature cheddar
- 50g parmesan (or vegetarian alternative), plus extra to top
- nutmeg , grated
- 50g gruyère or comté
- 1 tsp white wine vinegar or lemon juice

Directions:

1. Heat oven to 220C/200 fan/gas 9. Toss the cauliflower florets, leaves and sliced core with 1 tbsp olive oil in a roasting tin and season. Roast in the oven for 30-40 mins, or until the cauliflower is turning golden and smelling nutty. While it's roasting, heat 1 tbsp of olive oil in a non-stick frying pan and add the shallots, sugar and thyme. Cook for 10-15 mins until soft, sweet and caramelised. Add

the wine and cook for a few more mins until evaporated. Meanwhile, cook the pasta in salty boiling water until just cooked. Drain and set aside.

2. For the cheese sauce, melt the butter in a non-stick saucepan over a medium heat with the bay leaf. Add the flour and cook, stirring, for 2 mins or so, until the roux is starting to bubble. Pour in the milk, little by little, stirring with a whisk, until fully incorporated and you have a smooth, lump-free sauce. Cook for about 10 mins until thickened, and then season with nutmeg and black pepper. Next, add the cheese and stir over the heat until it's melted and smooth. Taste the sauce and adjust the seasoning, adding the vinegar or lemon juice to taste.

3. Tip the pasta and shallots into the cauliflower roasting dish, then pour over the cheese sauce and stir so everything is well coated. Sprinkle over the remaining parmesan, reduce the oven to 180C/160C fan/gas 4 and bake for 20 mins, or until golden. Remove from the oven and allow to settle for about 10 mins, then serve with a crisp chicory salad.

Lightning Source UK Ltd.
Milton Keynes UK
UKHW021128110521
383520UK00001B/67

9 781802 693607